Eft and Tapping

Use the Emotional Freedom Technique to De-stress

(Simple Diy Experiences to Prove That Your Mind Creates Your Life)

Liberty Barlowe

Published By **John Kembrey**

Liberty Barlowe

*Eft and Tapping: Use the Emotional Freedom
Technique to De-stress (Simple Diy Experiences to
Prove That Your Mind Creates Your Life)*

ISBN   978-1-998901-26-5

No part of this guidebook shall be reproduced in any form without permission in writing from the publisher except in the case of brief quotations embodied in critical articles or reviews.

Legal & Disclaimer

The information contained in this ebook is not designed to replace or take the place of any form of medicine or professional medical advice. The information in this ebook has been provided for educational & entertainment purposes only.

The information contained in this book has been compiled from sources deemed reliable, and it is accurate to the best of the Author's knowledge; however, the Author cannot guarantee its accuracy and validity and cannot be held liable for any errors or omissions. Changes are periodically made to this book. You must consult your doctor or get professional medical advice before using any of the suggested remedies, techniques, or information in this book.

Upon using the information contained in this book, you agree to hold harmless the Author from and against any damages, costs, and expenses, including any legal fees potentially resulting from the application of any of the information provided by this guide. This disclaimer applies to any damages or injury caused by the use and application, whether directly or indirectly, of any advice or information presented, whether for breach of contract, tort, negligence, personal injury, criminal intent, or under any other cause of action.

You agree to accept all risks of using the information presented inside this book. You need to consult a professional medical practitioner in order to ensure you are both able and healthy enough to participate in this program.

Table Of Contents

Introduction

You are about to find out precisely why we, as people, do what we do. Having studied human conduct for many years, I really have come to discover is that every one human beings react to troubles based totally on their emotions.

Therefore, if people permit their alternatives to be dominated with the useful resource of their emotions; we want to recognition on a manner to exchange how we experience to get what we need.

This is wherein tapping is to be had in, generally referred to as EFT. This stands for Emotional Freedom Technique. It is simplified as our inner machine of ideals; we make our lifestyles picks based totally on our very personal inner ideals.

The inner paradigm of ideals are constituted of past memories. These ideals are created and saved in your unconscious mind. All of your reports are recorded on your thoughts in conjunction with tastes, smells and recollections, for use for future reference.

As we cross about our every day life our selections can be primarily based totally on past memories and the feelings which is probably related to the ones reminiscences. These will then make contributions in developing our behavior. These may be each pinnacle or terrible conduct.

Unlike conventional EFT which makes use of meridian points at the same time as tapping, The Faster Tapping Method will produce longer lasting effects. After many years of everyday EFT I determined that I wasn't mission lasting effects. It wasn't till I positioned The Faster Tapping Method that everything changed for me.

I need to share this technique with you. I take transport of as genuine with it's going to assist you to gain any vicinity of your existence. I did no longer need this to be some one of a kind lengthy and stupid e book on the data of EFT. I designed this ebook to be a quick guide.

People are very busy within the present day day with many responsibilities and obligations. I want this to be a quick guide; one as a way to get at once to the point and of end result.

I will go over what you want to understand in vicinity of the whole thing there is to understand about The Faster Tapping Method. This way you can start to get fast results in recent times.

So capture a cup of coffee, sit down again and loosen up. You will fast examine the manner you can start to tap expand free.

Chapter 1: Eft-The Fundamentals

EFT is an tremendous restoration method, this is just like acupuncture thoughts except it doesn't rent needles as is completed in acupuncture. The approach has been confirmed as powerful in a huge style of issues associated with fitness, emotion, and performance. More often EFT has delivered approximately terrific and sturdy remedy in instances wherein special remedy modalities failed.

EFT—A brief history

Emotional Freedom Technique is effective in putting off the negative feelings that prevent you from reaching fulfillment in all elements of your existence. This technique is an electricity remedy based mostly on using meridian elements.

Developed thru Gary Craig from the direction breaking discoveries accomplished by means of Dr. Roger

Callahan, the method allows deal with numerous problems you face in life on the emotional and bodily diploma. Depression, headache, pain, phobias, addictive cravings, abandonment, nightmares, guilt, tension, anger, disturbing issues, and loads of various issues had been efficaciously handled with the technique.

Roger Callahan a Psychologist determined EFT by means of twist of fate, at the same time as he have become treating a affected individual, Mary, who modified into suffering from water phobia. Mary's phobia avoided her from acting her each day sports activities activities. She emerge as afraid even to energy nearby the ocean, and terrified each time it rained. Even the sight of water advanced her fear. The worry introduced on excessive emotional and bodily pain.

Dr. Callahan, who were analyzing about traditional remedies utilized by the Chinese, discovered out approximately electricity meridians. He have become inspired via the meridians and determined to try it out on Mary. He requested Mary to faucet on her cheekbone in which the stomach meridian factor become gift. The tapping delivered on a direct and splendid trade in Mary. The belly pain disappeared or even more high-quality turned into that her phobia for water too vanished. From this revelation, Dr. Callahan began out severa investigations on developing and perfecting the approach, which he named as Thought Field Therapy.

Under Dr. Callahan's steerage, Gary Craig professional in TFT. Later he advanced EFT after he found issues in the usage of the Thought Field Therapy techniques. EFT is a simplified and extra model formed from Callahan's approach.

EFT includes an clean to conform with collection of tapping elements for any kind of state of affairs. This has made it pretty well-known with folks that locate tapping an powerful manner to dispose of their emotional and physical ailments. Over the years for the motive that approach has been brought, tapping practitioners have carried out the strategies in complex and tough situations, and located the technique mainly a achievement

What does EFT contain?

Emotional Freedom Technique moreover termed as EFT tapping, or tapping, is a powerful recuperation tool used universally. It offers extremely good treatment in issues related to bodily and emotional health, and performance problems.

EFT is primarily based on the precept that irrespective of the type of improvement you are seeking out for your existence, the emotional issues determined in you, are the principle purpose for the issues you face. Emotional strain prevents natural restoration electricity of your frame even in case of chronic pain, diagnosed conditions, or physical issues.

While bodily signs and symptoms get relieved with out trouble without the want to find out the emotional causative factors, if you are looking for lengthy-time period results, it is important to recognize the related emotional problems and aim them

EFT moreover goals at achieving emotional freedom and piece to your existence with the assist of the Personal Peace Procedure. This strategies pastimes at vanquishing all self-proscribing beliefs, boosting personal performance, assist construct relationships and acquire suitable bodily fitness.

In a nutshell, EFT is an evolving technique you may use to clean away all emotional problems of your beyond and welcome the new traumatic situations in lifestyles with a inexperienced, healthful and tremendous mind-set.

Powerful benefits

EFT brings you the best of Chinese energy meridian method. While acupressure and acupuncture reputation on alleviating physical ache, EFT is going deeper and treats emotional problems, which may be the premise cause of all, bodily, emotional and not unusual usual overall performance associated problems you face in lifestyles. EFT and tapping gives a powerful mixture of bodily blessings discovered in acupuncture with cognitive advantages decided in traditional remedy techniques foremost to an all-encompassing and faster remedy.

Although EFT is connected to acupuncture, it differs in the way it brings about healing effect. EFT includes important modes of motion in particular

•   Connect mentally to the ideal issues you are affected with

•   Stimulate the concerned meridian elements through tapping with fingertips

9

When completed within the right manner, EFT lets in to balance the disturbances located in power elements or meridian points within the body. This permits to heal issues, which in any other case take a long time to heal. And most importantly the Tapping technique may be very clean to grasp and you can do it in any vicinity for your very own with notable results. Even kids can revel in the method.

Energy circuits in body

The Chinese round 5,000 years again decided an power circuit tool that spreads all over the frame. The circuits or meridians form the essential center of fitness practices in Eastern treatment and are the idea for acupuncture and acupressure, and remarkable treatment techniques.

When you faucet at the numerous meridian or electricity factors in conjunction with your fingertips, you may revel in profound modifications for your health each physical and emotionally.

Chapter 2: Get Faster Results

One of the numerous topics human beings will say is that they've been doing the tapping method and claim to now not be getting higher results.

The factor you want to go through in thoughts with tapping is that it's miles a talent. It is a existence talent. It is a lifestyles changing transformational manner.

Tapping works with the regulation of enchantment. The law of enchantment approach clearly, you attraction to some factor you dominantly cognizance on. Not what you think about a few times it's far your predominate thoughts that shape your reality.

So in case you are struggling to fix an problem, then that sincerely method that there are opinions and memories that you are not aware of and are holding at once to.

You need to increase your degree of awareness to famend what you're virtually maintaining at once to.

And the first-class way to do this is to get yourself a magazine and expand the addiction of journaling your horrible reminiscences and also to record all the outstanding reviews you've got had.

If you are making it a dependancy to popularity on first-class the best, it's going to begin to deliver greater true into your lifestyles. Because what you attention on will increase and increase.

I recognize that is straightforward stuff. But it's miles doing the fundamentals constantly over a long term that allows you to get you better effects.

If you are uncertain of what is retaining you once more, you then definately must ask yourself higher questions with enough intensity that your thoughts will have no preference but to provide you an answer.

Ask realistic questions that will help you circulate ahead quicker.

For example in case you ask: "Why cannot I get some element right?"

Your mind will offer you with the first issue it is aware about which might be: "Because you're dumb."

That isn't the shape of response that you need. You need responses a remarkable manner to supply higher solutions. And you do this through the use of manner of asking questions that allows you to offer you with higher answers to remedy your trouble.

For instance, if you need to shed pounds and recognize that it isn't so a laugh in losing weight and cannot discover the money for gym club, you may ask questions alongside the strains of:

This form of question will give you a better response.

If the answer does no longer come proper away keep asking the question with conviction and intensity and in the end the answer will come. It has to.

The first-rate way to get whatever particular on your lifestyles is to alternate the inner references to your thoughts.

By journaling, it'll help to search around exactly what it's far that is bothering you.

Then start tapping on the sensation. What many people do incorrect is that they wait till the problem gets to a far extra quantity.

You have to increase the addiction of tapping within the warmth of the right away.

Do now not wait till the reminiscence is saved away for future years. Tap and get free now. So the system is straightforward.

Get a magazine and write down every bad and excessive first-rate research.

Begin to faucet away the bad reports and maintain the brilliant reminiscences to take a look at even as instances get hard.

How do you recognize which feeling and reminiscence is right and that is awful? You will apprehend by the use of the usage of the manner you revel in. Your feelings will tell you.

Just ask yourself the way you sense approximately a selected memory. And decide if it is right or awful.

When life receives hard you could constantly circulate lower once more and feature a observe over your wonderful recollections. This will boom a spirit of gratitude, a good way to exchange your emotional u.S. Of america right right right into a wonderful kingdom.

The problem humans have at the same time as troubles upward push up is they forget about all the right that has befell to them inside the past and top notch consciousness at the bad.

With a magazine you'll constantly have this powerful tool, allowing you to refer yet again to and get your self in a higher emotional u . S . A ..

What is in the long run going that will help you alternate is creating a real fantastic choice. A real desire wherein you may be actually devoted to live with it regardless of what. Many humans make exceptional short picks.

Make up for your thoughts that you are going to constantly keep tapping till you get yourself in a higher emotional usa.

And when you have a difficult time growing a tough choice, then start tapping on that emotion. And then verify the brand new addiction you need to make bigger.

Chapter 3: Superficial Tapping

I strongly accept as true with there's a place for 'moderate' tapping. As with a few thing new, or used sporadically, a addiction hasn't been superior. Coupled with unconscious and aware resistance, this will and regularly does lead human beings to surrender early or no longer bypass deeper. That's on occasion wherein the "Tapping doesn't paintings"

or

"

I

'm a tapping failure" ideals originate.

Superficial tapping can paintings splendidly in lots of situations, and occasionally that's the splendid we are able to choice for for a while.

I become out with a chum whose vehicle emerge as extra dirt than metal. I commented that there has been a drive-via vehicle wash close by and why didn't we offer the car the as soon as-over there? She surely started out out shaking in truth on the idea. Car washes freak her out. Seriously, in the space of a few seconds she had prolonged beyond from cushty and happy to a '

7

' at the SUDs scale.

We stopped to get a drink and for her to clean her head a hint. Knowing I faucet (she's every other '

Fallen Angel

' who used to faucet however doesn't anymore) she changed into open to the idea, so we tapped down on her immediately tension. We didn't dig deeper into the motive, but definitely stored it mild and targeted on the immediately pain. By the time our liquids arrived she'd tapped all the manner down to zero, a span of in all likelihood less than mins.

I didn't press the issue, due to the fact a part of the '

art work

' of EFT is knowing even as to shut up. Phobias may be continual if there's a near cause, but many phobias, like fear of car washes or clowns or pterodactyls are fairly situational and in large detail avoidable.

She volunteered the data that the lack of manage emerge as a large part of her automobile wash fear. Being 'trapped' inside the automobile and at the '

mercy

' of the cascades of water and the machines. Then, a few component of an belief. She said she stopped tapping due to the same element. That she may hit an artery, lose manage, and not be able to get it again.

More insights: she never goes to places wherein she feels she may be trapped, like movie theatres, ships and boats, and on planes and public transport. She's no longer socially demanding or pretty strung. It's just the concern of no longer having an break out route that devices her off.

That second while you in fact witness a person going from fear to willpower. "

We

're going through the car wash. Now." She stated it, no longer me. I advised infant steps. There come to be no critical important to undergo the wash.

We went through the automobile wash in baby steps. Arriving, we tapped down the growing anxiety earlier than we were given out of the car to pay. Then we tapped after paying but earlier than committing to the get admission to. From the get entry to and all of the way thru the showering approach we tapped, focused handiest on 'This demanding feeling', which at some level in the machine in no manner rose above '

2

'. Remember that it come to be a '

7

' at the equal time as, numerous kilometres earlier and now not a automobile wash in sight, she perception about it.

That's whilst situational tapping comes into its very very own. It doesn't searching out to find out and cope with the center problem, best to alleviate the on the spot and obvious symptoms.

Superficial tapping is unique. It's tapping spherical the rims of a hassle with out getting towards any proper belief into what's the use of it. Unfortunately, the upward thrust of the 'sound chunk' on the Internet encourages and helps this.

The very modern-day nature of the tap-along is like the overall nature of karaoke. You don't need to learn how to have a examine the song; you clearly need to have a have a look at the activates, repeat the traces, and apprehend the overall track. It's the tapping equal of 'swing your associate dosey doe'

.

It calls for some diploma of self-analysis, with out a bargain initial or ongoing research into what the real troubles can be. In this tool, tapping down current symptoms replaces a radical investigation.

Your symptoms and signs and symptoms are quietened however you basically live the same. This is not the liberty implied in the EFT name.

You got here to tapping for a purpose. Something each wasn't proper or wasn't present. It can be that every one your problems had been consequences regular but, given that you're studying this, it's a stable bet they haven't been. I suspect that very regularly unconscious resistance is the culprit, arriving prolonged in advance than someone honestly is aware of enough about tapping as a manner to recognize and conquer it.

The mass of records handy may be overwhelming. In the growing body of statistics that's been accrued and collated during the last two a long time, and similarly overlaid with opinion quantities, podcasts, YouTube movement photographs, mailing lists, books, CDs, publications, and so forth,

the selection can turn out to be the hassle

.

Simplify, commit, use. It's that clean and that tough. It'll take you to places you'd as an possibility no longer bypass, however it'll additionally take you to wherein you want to be.

Another avoidable problem is the self-created one. It takes location while you try to pressure yourself into an wrong or incomplete forestall. I've decided it to be noticeably common.

Back in 1999 I decided to paintings on a big problem. In tapping, we're advised to appearance what comes up and take a look at it (chase the ache) or as a minimum write it down for later reference. My mom came up often, however by way of way of and huge at quite low stages. However, I happy myself that quantity become extra critical than great, if you realize what I propose. Fifteen '

4

's are extra than '

nine

,

s.

One of my brothers every so often got here up, too, however I dismissed his importance due to the fact we were in no way near. See how the rational mind casts the number one caregiver due to the fact the villain, and the a long way flung brother as certainly an worrying bit player?

With the benefit of experience and hindsight, I'd say my unconscious resistance was at art work, kidding me proper into a secure area of no ache, no gain, however frequently no pain, in preference to pushing me into the actual ache and out the opportunity element to freedom and contentment.

After a few months of tapping at the trouble and genuinely getting very little out of it, my brother came to mind and I decided in frustration to examine that notion and take a look at what need to arise. Well, explosive rage is what came about. I've in no manner been that angry in my life, in advance than or considering the truth that.

It modified into fantastic.

All of a sudden torrents of stuff have been surfacing, a lot of them with immoderate emotional pain connected. The quantity of '

9

's and '

10

's I registered could have torn the planet aside if they'd been earthquakes. This went on for the best a part of a month. I actually have become withdrawn, sullen, and without troubles delivered on. Fortunately, and this is vital for you, too ...

I didn't take it out on others

.

Please, do no longer go to damage and wreckage onto others, whether or not or not you realize them or now not. Those human beings may not have the information and advantage of tapping, and also you don't want to be including new guilt, anger, and disenchanted while you're searching for to lessen them in different troubles.

I suspect quite a few EFT promoters don't communicate about those effects due to the reality they don't need to place people off the usage of EFT. I don't have an answer for you on that. If you're a parent, have a large other, responsibilities at artwork, home, or in the community, I can't glibly tell you it'll be all right and to truely soldier on. Maybe you can't manage to pay for a retreat wherein you can 'get it completed'. I recognize there have been times as quickly as I couldn't discover the coins for to breathe.

Perhaps there aren't any practitioners (or top notch ones) on your area, or maybe there are however you could't find the money for one. I had one absolutely rubbish certified practitioner in my place lower back then and it changed into a whole waste of coins I need to have better utilized by paying in area of delaying a few bills.

The first-rate I can tell you is that I haven't for my part noted everybody who doesn't have at the least one big hassle, and normally there are more. The ultimate man or woman I helped before hollering 'enough' changed into as I defined above. A mother, a associate, a begin-up businesswoman, confused to the eyeballs, and without enough cash to take a month off to lease a lovely cabin within the woods and thru the lake.

She knew a number of her biggies and we discovered some extra. We advanced a plan that could be a 365 days in the execution. Instead of undertaking too deeply and tearing everything out right away, we 'peeled the onion' at a gradual pace. It labored fantastically. It took dedication, due to the fact lots is going on in a year and the results aren't commonly instantaneous and apparent, however it worked.

You want to discover some form of hard balance among getting it carried out and giving up as it's taking too lengthy. You've lived in conjunction with your stuff this lengthy. Commit to a yr of unloading it, peacefully however absolutely.

Let

's appearance now at how ridiculous our mantra is turning into.

"Tapping doesn't art work for me." Are you still as positive as you as soon as had been?

"Tapping stopped going for walks." Did you get even the smallest restart inside the direction of any of this ebook?

"EFT doesn't paintings." Have you attempted a few brilliant procedures to help you get going once more?

"

I

'm an EFT failure." I don't remember you. And I in no way will. You've in all likelihood honestly picked up some terrible behavior or statistics or data. Use tapping to assist alternate them.

Chapter 4: Frequently Occurring Blockages That Save You Economic Success

When it consists of coins specially, a commonplace bad belief that many humans preserve is that they do no longer sincerely need to be rich. Like such pretty a few wonderful beliefs this may occasionally lurk under the ground far from conscious be aware. They may additionally need to be rich, however deep down sense that they do not surely deserve it.

Another not unusual blockage relates to a fear of resentment for having cash. This fear frequently starts out as resentment itself: resentment for rich people along side celebrities, lottery winners, or maybe pals, accomplice and youngsters, or buddies who display as plenty as have extra cash. When a person resents distinctive people for being wealthier than they he is, he is probably aware of his resentment as it exists largely "above the floor". However what he won't perceive so without problem is the worry of being resented with the aid of the use of others if he himself want to ever be financially a success. This fear can fester and boom through the years, subsequently becoming loads greater debilitating than the genuine resentment that brought on it. This is a superb example of the way living on negativity handiest serves to draw similarly negativity into our lives.

The backside line, with regards to monetary achievement is that whether or now not we advantage it or now not relies upon to a totally massive diploma on our blockages that relate to coins. If we aren't making enough cash it's miles likely related to our a few blockage that we've were given have been for the reason that we may not be aware of. Even if we're making enough money but just spending too much of it, this too is regularly associated with a blockage. Lots of people, after they start making loads of cash after a length of being horrible, or unexpectedly come into money, together with prevailing the lottery or having a business organisation assignment abruptly take off, sabotage themselves and their success. This is shockingly common with lottery winners. They do now not understand themselves as being wealthy people, they do no longer need the responsibility of being rich, they be by way of one of the blockages we've were given discussed above, or a few different blockage. Whatever the case may be, research recommend that an amazingly excessive percentage of folks that win the lottery are once more to the identical monetary scenario they were in previous to winning the lottery inner best three years of triumphing. The strategies the ones lottery winners lose their cash varies. They might also deliver it away, make investments it poorly, spend it on opulent and vain conspicuous consumption items, or locate other techniques to cut up themselves from it. Whatever their movements can be, the idea purpose of these times is certainly usually a few form of blockage, generally a blockage that the person become no longer even privy to.

Chapter 5: How Eft Works On Your Body?

Every day you stumble upon numerous reviews which your thoughts catalogues and stores, often connected with an emotion. Your mind constantly takes in statistics from the encompassing global and deletes facts deemed beside the point. When you pay interest a particular call (for instance, a terrible ex) your thoughts will look for this facts and retrieve records along thing the emotion associated with him/her. Studies have observed that humans are capable of undergo in mind terrible events hundreds quicker than happier ones. This is probably way the idea of an ex (especially a contemporary one) want to damage a beautifully appropriate day.

As defined in advance than, on the equal time because the mind retrieves awful activities it additionally consists of horrible emotions with it, say fear, anger and so on. These awful reports moreover transmit an alert message to brain within the form of electrical impulses that would bring about imbalance or blockage, which paves the manner to emotional and physical troubles.

EFT works by way of the use of tapping energy meridian factors at the body while citing excessive satisfactory statements in case you need to "reprogram" the ones terrible reviews into fine ones. This approach requires handiest the pointers of your fingers to yield the famous great response for your frame. Kinetic energy can be transferred to the ones meridians at the same time as you're concerned or stressful about a selected problem and at which trouble you will need to country high great statements to dam the terrible strength. This exercise helps to retrain your meridian device and exchange the bad energy proper right into a exceptional one.

When do you need to do tapping?

The solution is simple, do it as frequently as you can, so that you can enjoy the advantages of tapping on your each day existence. I suggest at the least 3 times an afternoon and you may do it yet again at the equal time as terrible feelings start to flare up. You can also even do that on the equal time as you're in public locations, say in case you are prepared in the airport for the flight or if you are enjoyable at your table.

Meridians

All strong items are made from electricity, so is your body. Medical checks like electroencephalography(EEG) or a magnetic resonance imaging (MRI) test will let you diploma this. Picture your body as a 3d roadmap, you must be able to without problem visualize a complete network of paths intersecting each extraordinary like electric circuits. This is what meridians are. These electrical circuits are energy assets hyperlink to every atom, cellular and organ to your body. These energy meridians additionally interconnect with each other and deliver facts at awesome speeds. If your emotional fitness is proper and properly balanced, those meridians preserve correct stability and this is useful on your commonplace properly-being.

There are particular energy meridians which can be as follows:

• Lung Meridian

• Colon Meridian

• Stomach Meridian

• Spleen Meridian

• Heart Meridian

• Intestine Meridian

• Pericardium Meridian

• Bladder Meridian

• Triple Warmer Meridian

- Kidney Meridian

- Gall Bladder Meridian

- Liver Meridian

Tapping on those meridian elements help to transmit vibrations throughout your frame which permits to rebalance the power tool.

Scientific Research

Whenever a brand new clinical remedy is first added, people are rightfully skeptical approximately it and the consequences it guarantees. Ever because the advent of EFT, there has been masses of studies done to affirm the effectiveness of this treatment.

A assessment have become published inside the magazine titled Review of General Psychology, which found out that EFT continuously exhibited high top notch results whilst coupled with clinical remedies in comparison to scientific treatment on my own.

A comparable observe turned into done on sixteen teenage boys who had records of bodily or intellectual abuse. They had been capable of cope masses better with the worrying recollections after they had completed a unmarried EFT session.

Another test have become finished on thirty depressed college students. The organisation that acquired EFT treatment, which crafted from about six hours, displayed decrease levels of despair after they were evaluated after 3 weeks.

A take a look at undertaken with the aid of the Iraq Vets Stress Project furthermore validates the overall performance of EFT and tapping. The have a look at changed into executed on hundred veterans who be afflicted by means of immoderate PTSD. Ninety percent of the vets have been certainly healed from the consequences of PTSD after taking in reality 6 instructions that lasted for 1 hour each. To make sure the effectiveness of

EFT and tapping, they accomplished each distinct take a look at at the equal company after 3 months, which observed out that the signs of PTSD were although lengthy long gone.

A precise have a have a look at modified into accomplished to discover the possibility of the usage of EFT in the treatment of immoderate depth headaches, which moreover confirmed top notch consequences. Frequency and depth of complications had been significantly decreased for the sufferers who practiced the EFT technique often.

EFT has additionally helped to reduce the strain hormones (degree of cortisol) notably in humans. A test was completed via a good mag in the United States, Journal of Nervous and Mental disorder. The studies confirmed that EFT helped to lessen the cortisol stages thru 24% in individuals who practiced EFT.

Another observe have become finished to determine the effectiveness of EFT within the remedy of human beings suffering from phobias of small animals and bugs, which moreover proved to be effective. Individuals who practiced EFT confirmed a much extra bargain inside the signs and symptoms and signs in their phobias in evaluation to folks who used awesome the deep studying method.

A look at accomplished via Dr. Swingle showed that EFT is likewise an powerful treatment, that could treatment individuals stricken by epilepsy. Kids who have been affected by epilepsy had been furnished with EFT therapy with the useful resource of using their dad and mom whenever the dad and mom suspected that there was a hazard for his or her epilepsy to be triggered. The have a have a study moreover observed exceptional and steady consequences for long-time period remedy.

Hopefully this financial ruin has furthermore eliminated any skepticism you may have had. There are also numerous resources at the net and other research that assist spotlight the performance and effectiveness of this technique. In the subsequent financial ruin I will teach you a way to surely do EFT. This consists of a manner to find out proper tapping points and tapping scripts.

A particular example of an EFT setup script that you may use if you be afflicted with the useful resource of depression might be "Even although I currently be stricken through despair, I take shipping of that I may be able to overcome this case and do well in my lifestyles".

Depression Script

After you've got got completed tapping and reciting your setup word like "Even even though I enjoy depressed, I take delivery of the manner I revel in and nevertheless love myself" you may use the following script for tapping in location of the use of the reminder word. Of direction for it to be greater effective you want to replace the sentences at the side of your private mind and emotions.

EFT Round 1: Express the Depression

Top of the top   This disappointment that I actually have

Eyebrow Is difficult to live with

Side of the attention   It makes me revel in hopeless

Under the attention   It absolutely wears me down

Under the nose   It makes everything seem colourless

Chin It's sapping my strength

Collar bone And draining my happiness

Under the arm   It's difficult to open up about it

EFT Round 2: Understand the Depression

Top of the pinnacle   What is inflicting this feel?

Eyebrow What is the supply?

Side of the eye   Why is it affecting me?

Under the attention   This melancholy

Under the nostril   Is robbing me of my happiness

Chin And positivity

Collar bone It's not serving me

Under the arm   How can I restoration it?

EFT Round 3: Explore the possibilities

Top of the top   I want to appearance the best in existence

Eyebrow And open myself as a first rate deal as genuine possibilities

Side of the eye   With each my mind and my coronary heart

Under the attention   Even if subjects sense hard to do

Under the nostril   They receives plenty less difficult with time

Chin If I can alternate my recognition and thoughts-set

Collar bone To a greater wonderful outcome

Under the arm   Then I can live life extra honestly

EFT Round four: Opening Up

Top of the pinnacle   I'm willing

Eyebrow To pay attention and attempt new subjects

Side of the eye   I'm inclined

Under the attention   To skip on with my lifestyles

Under the nose   And leave this disappointment behind me

Chin It serves no cause

Collar bone It pleasant drains me

Under the arm   My future may be colourful yet again

EFT Round five: Choosing Confidence and Hopefulness

Top of the top   I choose out to launch this terrible strength

Eyebrow And to cognizance on a superb very last consequences

Side of the eye   When I permit pass of this sadness and negativity

Under the eye   I turns into extra assured and hopeful

Under the nose   When I'm assured and hopeful

Chin I becomes re-energized with existence again

Collar bone This positivity and energy will replace my depression

Under the arm   I will live a notable and satisfied lifestyles

Chapter 6: How Eft Works

The emotional freedom approach uses acupressure and psychology to assist enhance a person's emotional fitness. Even notion emotional fitness has a tendency to be ignored, it plays a critical issue in a person's bodily fitness and their capability to heal. It doesn't rely how committed someone is to maintaining right way of life and weight loss plan, in the occasion that they have got emotional boundaries reputation of their way, they received't accumulate the body that they want.

Most of the time, you could observe EFT right now for your bodily symptoms and signs and signs to find out remedy without jogging through the emotional people. However, for a effective and lasting stop result, you need to determine out and artwork thru the emotional troubles.

The premise of EFT additionally is conscious that the more emotional troubles you may work through, the greater emotional peace and freedom you may have. With EFT you could cast off limiting ideals, increase private typical overall performance, decorate relationships, and function higher physical fitness. To be sincere, everybody on Earth has a couple of emotional issues that they'll be maintaining onto.

EFT is fantastically clean to investigate and could permit you to in regions which embody: task effective desires, eliminating or lessen pain, discount of food cravings, and the elimination of horrible emotions. And that's definitely the start of what it may do for you.

EFT is based totally absolutely at the meridians of power which have been applied in traditional acupuncture to heal emotional and bodily issues for introduced than 5 thousand years, but with out the use of needles. Instead, it makes use of smooth tapping of the fingertips to transport kinetic power into a specific meridian on the identical time as you reflect onconsideration on your trouble and talk an affirmation.

The use of affirmations and tapping the meridians help to easy the emotional block from the bioenergy machine. This then permits to repair the body and mind balance this is wanted for optimum tremendous health.

There are many which can be cautious of this workout before the whole thing, mainly the mind of electromagnetic energy that flows through the body. Then are others which is probably bowled over by using the mind of the manner EFT tapping works.

To begin EFT, there are matters that you need to apprehend: the tapping elements and the strategies. We will check the technique proper right here and the tapping elements in a while in the e-book.

You want to recognize that with this method you'll be tapping together collectively along with your fingers. There are numerous acupuncture meridians that live in your fingertips, so whilst you tap, you're the use of the electricity in your fingertips in addition to the energy of the vicinity that you are tapping.

Traditionally the tapping is finished with the beneficial resource of the index and center finger and with one hand nice. You can use whichever hand that you need. Many of the tapping elements are on either aspect of your frame, so meaning you may use whichever facet you want, and you could transfer sides inside the path of a tapping consultation.

You can also adjust the exercise via using all your hands and each fingers to create a mild, natural curved line. The greater hands you use, them more acupuncture factors you could get right of access to to. You may also even cowl extra region so that you can hit the factors simpler than with multiple arms. It's additionally critical which you take off any bracelets or watches that you will be carrying.

Affirmation Statements

Another crucial element is developing with the confirmation announcement that you will use. Traditionally, the word is some aspect like "Even idea I sincerely have this (fill inside the smooth), I deeply and without a doubt get hold of myself."

You would probably fill inside the clean with a short description of the terrible emotion, food yearning, addiction, or different trouble that you are experiencing.

You can also use the following variations. All of the subsequent are tremendous to use because of the truth they use the equal essential format. Meaning, they famend what the trouble is and create popularity no matter the hassle's lifestyles. Those are the topics which can be vital in growing an effective confirmation. The traditional one is a great deal less tough to keep in mind, however experience unfastened to apply one of the following.

"I accept myself notwithstanding the truth that I (fill in the smooth)," or "Even notwithstanding the fact that I (fill inside the easy), I profoundly and deeply take shipping of myself."

You can also use "I receive and love myself even though I (fill inside the clean)."

Some interesting statistics approximately affirmations are:

You do now not ought to hold in mind you confirmation actually; all you have to do is say it.

It's extra powerful if you may say it with emphasis and feeling, however in reality announcing it'll but do the hobby.

It's higher to talk it out loud, but if you are in public where you want to mutter it or do it silently, it's miles going to be simply as effective.

You can tune into your hassle surely by using the usage of thinking of what it's miles.

If you don't song into your hassle, which creates energy disruptions, then EFT will now not be powerful.

Advice and Caution

You want to great ever do what feels proper for yours. Never enter into any bodily or emotional waters that could be threatening. It's your device to make certain you stay solid in this putting. You can effortlessly are seeking out professional help in case you want to. Here is a few recommendation in advance than you dive into EFT.

• It is extraordinarily important that you are exquisite precise collectively in conjunction with your language on the same time as you use EFT

• You ought to be completely tuned into your trouble. Many instances, if you are coping with some factor that is very painful, you can attempt to disconnect from your feelings.

• Because you are strolling with energy, it's miles essential to pay interest for a cognitive shift. You will recognize when one has happened due to the reality you may reframe the hassle. When you see the problem from a certainly one of a kind mind-set, you could probable be amazed or have a present day perception. This is great at the same time as this happens, and it could open new, valuable insights.

• Make great you stay well hydrated. Water allows to behavior electricity, and you're gaining access to electric powered powered power while jogging in the path of EFT.

EFT Application Range

The only element which can limit what EFT can do for you is your creativeness. Experienced practitioners and the EFT originators all around the global, among them, are psychotherapists and psychologists, have used EFT on numerous incredible troubles. This manner that have used not first-rate with emotional problems, wherein it works the brilliant but for distinct physical troubles, with brilliant success on every occasion there's an emotional detail or traumatic studies.

But that's no longer the most effective element; EFT is also a exquisite device to use for non-public improvement. It can assist to dispose of self-imposed rules that prevent people from experiencing abundance, extremely good relationships, wealth, and happiness of their life.

In EFT's brief information, it has already been able to assist over one thousand people with many commonplace emotional problems, collectively with:

• Confusion, grief, guilt and almost each different emotion you can trust, collectively with the yucky, icky, and awful emotions that you may't call

• Self-doubt

• Inner little one troubles and horrible memories

• All styles of phobias and fears

• Depression

• Frustration and anger

• Anxiety and strain

The top notch thing is that the benefits don't cease there. EFT tapping isn't in reality restrained to doing away with painful emotions.

1. Better health:

a. Increases someone's standard nicely-being

b. Helps insomnia

c. Pain remedy

d. The cut fee of physical cravings for things like cigarettes and chocolate

2. Better effectiveness in the matters which you do:

a. Speak inside the the front of a crown and with the people that you are not capable of communicate with within the interim

b. Better private and organisation relationships

c. Get rid of barriers approximately cash and open yourself as a lot as growing abundance to your lifestyles

d. Improve how you perform in sports, venture, and each other areas of your lifestyles

e. Grow your possibilities in your profession

three. Make your first-rate of life better

a. Improve you spiritual and personal growth

b. Create greater braveness to attempt things that you have desired to, however have been afraid to

c. Get rid of any feelings that maintain you from having a lifestyles the is whole of love and joy

There are many examples of human beings that have been capable of with out problems get over feelings that have them for years, and sometimes a few years, with the usage of EFT. It has been something that humans might also want to turn to for assist even as not anything else has been capable of help them. It has moreover efficiently helped reduce several physical structures along side insomnia, again ache, and complications.

The strength of EFT is at its wonderful at the equal time because the bodily signs and symptoms are also related to tension and strain. The builders of EFT had said a success rate of eighty to a hundred percent even as it came to emotional troubles. When it includes physical illnesses, the share of fulfillment is genuinely decrease. Most of the time, the effects of EFT are eternal and inside the occasion that they aren't you could with out problems repeat the manner if desired.

It works quick and is moderate. Often human beings can release feelings like stress, anger, tension, and fear in a unmarried session, a few days, or multiple weeks in comparison to months or years even because it comes to traditional remedy.

One of the first-class things approximately EFT is the truth that it is so bendy. When you grasp the competencies that it takes, which aren't difficult, it's miles nearly like growing your superpowers. You can use the ones tools in pretty lots any situation. Like if you have a big presentation to offer at paintings, or you're stepping into for a method interview, you could use EFT proper in advance than to help relax out your anxiety. It does no longer require some thing precise, but it certainly works wonders and can be used anywhere.

Chapter 7: The Basics Of Mindfulness: Discovering What Your Mind Can Do

The well-known announcing "What your mind can conceive, your frame can benefit" has been notably used in order to encourage people to pursue some thing their cause is. This is because of the truth if their mind is ready on a single goal, the frame may be directed as to what actions need to be taken to reap it. Fortunately, this announcing is likewise relevant in assisting us cope with troubles and invite fantastic vibes in our life.

This economic damage goals to discover the fundamentals of mindfulness – what it's miles, and the manner its workout can cause a higher life.

What is mindfulness?

Mindfulness is a form of meditation which pursuits to become privy to your emotions, sensations, and mind while you are in a non-judgmental and relaxed kingdom. In a much less difficult experience, its aim is to apprehend what's happening with your self internally and inside the present 2d. When a person is conscious, they will be capable of see the whole thing spherical them sincerely, and aren't worried with what or how topics have to be.

Mindfulness is stated to be similar to a Buddhist meditation practiced which have end up started out round 2500 years in the beyond. However, mindfulness isn't a religiously related meditation technique, and all people regardless of their non secular affiliation can exercise it.

A majority of the time, our mind capabilities on vehicle pilot at the same time as we cross about our every day actions. This is a very green tool that the mind uses. However, so often we discover ourselves behaving in strategies that don't line up with what we fee. I'm constantly caught in the trap of in which I realise I want to be and what I'm sincerely doing within the gift second. I get so irritated with myself even as my behaviors don't line up with my values. Why is it that I need to do "pinnacle", but I can't? When I don't want to do "terrible," I do it except? How stressful this cycle is for me.

Fortunately, the mind is wise and is privy to that it doesn't continuously get it proper. That's why it deliver us recognition so we're able to interrupt the manner and turn off the car pilot. Mindfulness is clearly the important factor to turning the auto pilot off and improving your functionality to apprehend what your thoughts is doing.

There are such quite a few extremely good benefits to mindfulness meditation. This is really a really interesting time for mindfulness and technological understanding. Research on the incredibleness of mindfulness is growing unexpectedly because of the truth scientists are understanding how pivotal mindfulness is on our mind fitness. It acquired't be long in advance than mindfulness sky rockets via the populace and each person can be doing it. It's form of like how yoga have become well-known and little yoga studios popped up anywhere. In the same way, I take delivery of as proper with that mindfulness may be taught in faculties and there additionally can be studios doping up across the metropolis. It turns into commonplace vicinity, because it want to.

Could you consider within the event that they in reality taught those devices in college? I'm a teacher so I get honestly fired up about this. I educate sensible lifestyles capabilities to my university college college students and now wherein within the curriculum is this form of beneficial and lifestyles changing functionality taught. If people had been educated on a manner to deal with stress, anger, melancholy, cravings, and so on, our international is probably any such one-of-a-kind region. Ooooh, it receives me excited at the possibilities of what might be. That's why this ebook is so crucial to me.

So what are its benefits?

The following benefits may be skilled through people who exercise mindfulness:

• It can help lower strain – utilizing mindfulness in each day conditions has been determined to lower pressure. When someone is within the usa of mindfulness, they may be more capable of decide the root cause of their problem. It may even help them to prioritize which hassle ought to be attended to first. As their mind turns into open to their troubles without poor thoughts, higher solutions can be conceived. Ultimately, this may result in solving the complete hassle.

• It can assist prevent depression and anxiety – some people are without problem crushed even as they are confronted with troubles that appear to stack one after some distinct. As you are able to prioritize which problems should be solved first thru utilizing mindfulness, the sensation that you may't get over them will in the end fade away. Similarly, the feeling of melancholy is also reduced. After all, the greater manipulate you've got with the state of affairs, the less annoying and the extra emotionally stable you're.

• It can assist beautify your physical fitness – it's far common for meditation methods to embody rest strategies. Deep respiratory and getting calm, a number of the behaviors decided in meditation strategies, are recognized to beautify coronary coronary heart rate and reduce blood strain.

• It can improve your memory and mental features – in particular, mindfulness can also beautify a person's memory. This is due to the fact mindfulness calls for you to don't forget every possible situation that you've professional during the day. You are also pressured to assume of each feasible technique to situations which may be causing you issues. As you operate your thoughts extra, your intellectual function will enhance as nicely. The way of mindfulness in reality rewires the thoughts. Studies at the mind display extraordinary enhancements to the mind in as brief as weeks!

• It permits you spot the situation on a present day day moderate – even the worst feasible state of affairs that you can ever bear in mind has a silver lining. Either there may be a meaning in the returned of it, or there may be a lesson that you can look at from it. With the help of mindfulness, it becomes less tough to see the problem in every special angle. This in turn will allow you to come to be extra incredible in managing the hassle and avoid having terrible feelings about it.

• It curbs your cravings – mindfulness practices had been used to control food cravings or maybe sturdy emotions. The SOBER approach, so that you can be shared later, is a top notch approach that comes out on pinnacle via research research on cravings.

• It builds self confidence and self recognition – mindfulness notices our mind for what they are: independent. There aren't any "right" or "terrible" mind. Just thoughts. The problem is at the same time as we display up and be part of which means to those thoughts. But mindfulness actually shall we those mind go with the flow thru our thoughts and now not attach which means to them. As fast as the ones mind come is as fast as they leave. I placed this concept profound and it genuinely clicked with me. Many years ago, when I become wrestling with post partum depression, I observed out approximately this concept in counseling. I so frequently may have bombarding thoughts that would go through my mind that I associated as poor. As a prevent end result, I may beat myself up for having those thoughts and label myself in horrible techniques. However, when I discovered out that I can in reality permit my mind pass thru my mind whilst no longer having any attachment to who I become as someone – I have become let loose! What a comfort for me. I hold to exercise this concept to this cutting-edge.

• It enhances power of will – strength of will is a key issue in the exceptional and duration of our existence. It behaves like a muscle that wants to get exercised so that you can increase huge. We all recognize that our lives is probably lots greater a success if we absolutely did the behaviors that we recognise we must. More frequently than not, we don't due to the fact we aren't disciplined enough to take a look at through. Consequently, we've developed a addiction of not doing rather than a addiction of doing. Mindfulness meditation is one of the quality procedures that you may considerably enhance your strength of will. Research studies show that the improvements to our thoughts are nearly immediate!

• It will growth your coronary heart rate variability – your coronary heart charge variability is connected in conjunction with your energy of thoughts. Science is likewise zeroing in its influences in our frame. So a long way, we recognize that our coronary coronary heart rate variability communicates how hundreds electricity of thoughts is at our disposal. Obviously, the wider our coronary coronary coronary heart price variability, the better our strength of thoughts can be. Meditation is one of the great techniques for reinforcing your coronary heart charge variability. The effects in studies are confirmed to be almost immediately. Again, I speak more about coronary coronary coronary heart charge variability, and what to do/now not do in

"Willpower." Another useful resource so as to use is www.Heartmath.Org. You really need to type in "coronary heart price variability" into their are in search of for engine.

Why mindfulness isn't always that easy?

Since mindfulness shares the identical practices decided in different meditation techniques, you may suppose that it isn't always that tough to use. This belief, however, is faux. This is because of the truth the following problems are professional by using way of way of folks who practice mindfulness:

• Some of your expectations might not be met — people who start utilizing mindfulness meditation usually have low expectancies in advance than the whole thing. But as they preserve to have interaction on this interest for pretty some time, their expectation of the prevalence of results will boom. After all, they've given enough time and opportunity for this method to reveal consequences, and it's far herbal for humans to assume results from a few element that they've spent their time on. Unfortunately, mindfulness isn't much like prescription medicine, because it in no way gives effects at once. Even if cause of mindfulness is to provide the advantages stated above, there can be no specific time table as to on the equal time as its effects can be professional. If expectancies aren't met, there is a huge tendency that the character will prevent meditating, with the notion that this technique "does now not work". Although you may no longer however see adjustments, recognise that your brain and heart chemistry proper away react, as verified through scans in the course of research.

• Its workout could make you experience uncomfortable – whilst a person starts meditation, they may both be bodily uncomfortable, or their thoughts may also moreover additionally purpose them soreness.

a. Being physical uncomfortable – in this shape of meditation, you are required to remain in a seated function or in different comfortable characteristic. However, getting uncomfortable can not be prevented, in particular if you have to maintain the said position for a sizeable amount of time. Although being aware about what your frame is experiencing can be a part of the routine, the ones problems may be considerable sufficient and can interrupt your meditation.

b. Getting uncomfortable collectively together along with your thoughts – while someone isn't in motion, his or her thoughts will carry into consciousness special mind or thoughts. Although having extra of those mind are beneficial in formulating answers on your troubles, the surge of thoughts can also create extra confusion as to that is the tremendous answer on your trouble. Simply positioned, it could slow down their tempo on the identical time as making alternatives. There also can be instances when undesirable mind ground due to the fact the meditation continues, which can emerge as distracting in the event that they study thru it. And despite the fact that the meditation emerge as stopped because of the non-save you re-surfacing of the unwanted idea, the reality that it modified into added into interest could make it tough that allows you to miss approximately it. There is a risk that you'll be adding every other hassle which you want to remedy.

Although it is able to be tough to start, it's essential to begin. Habits take at least 21 days to form. This is without a doubt a dependancy you want to shape! Start small on a each day foundation. Begin with 3 minutes and paintings your way as much as 1o or 15 mins or longer. Don't beat your self up in case you are not able to decide to 10 – 15 mins. It is higher to have a quick meditation exercising than none the least bit. You will nonetheless accumulate the profound blessings.

Chapter 8: Why Tapping Works

Tapping works because of the truth not handiest have authors and self-proclaimed practitioners boasted extraordinary effects, but because of the fact the method is based absolutely in sound historic proof.

Tapping is part intellectual, element physiological, or maybe trouble religious. In practices of medicine and psychology, the premise of the trouble is normally the supply at which to exchange your life-style. Either with reprogramming your mind to assume a excessive high-quality, more powerful, way or with changing your physical behavior to preserve you greater healthful, it is typically the most number one shape of our problems that have to be addressed. And in addressing them, our lives decorate.

The method of tapping does focus on the use of bodily stress factors in preference to deep-digging into issues of tension or past trauma, however the approach is sound: you need a clean and handy physical, actual-worldwide tool an terrific way to supply you toward your intellectual, emotional, and intellectual solution. If you don't have a ordinary, a mantra, or some thing to bodily do to resource your illnesses, you'd really be questioning your troubles, and the day, away.

This handiest creates more problems, as frequently we want a breather for our brains in order not to get over excited and to get closer to our results.

Tapping works because it gives you the physical reminder to refocus your mind, and also you're being attentive to your very personal voice out loud in preference to to your head. Additionally, the bodily touch is reassuring, and that comfort automatically alleviates our stressors, which opens the doorways for alternate.

And even as you open the door for exchange, particularly even as you had been able to inspire your self to do it on your personal, the opportunities will without a doubt be endless.

Chapter 9: Tapping Affirmations

Tapping, while properly administered, may be an excellent technique of relieving emotional troubles and pressure. The effect is much like many particular famous strategies like paying attention to calm and enjoyable song, speakme to a person approximately the hassle being experienced, and speakme calmly to at least one's very very very own self. However, no longer like those unique strategies, EFT will assist you cope with any emotional turmoil or lack of confidence of any type.

To gather maximum advantage from tapping you can also need to u . S . An affirmation as you faucet. Most EFT practitioners advise starting with the following:

"Even notwithstanding the truth that I truely have this _____, I deeply and sincerely accept myself."

This is called an EFT Setup Affirmation.

Self-reputation

Self-splendor is a distinctive feature that needs to be employed with the aid of manner of each and each one human beings. Resistance, or mental reversal, takes region whilst a part of us wants to exchange however some other component (usually an unconscious element), is proof in opposition to the exchange. Such resistance is taken into consideration considered one of the most important boundaries to achieving and preserving prolonged-time period achievement with the Emotional Freedom Technique.

One of the maximum commonplace sorts of resistance, or psychological reversal, is the disability to truely take transport of our self regardless of some issue fears or issues that we may be experiencing. On the alternative hand, while we resist or reject who we are and the scenario that we find ourselves in, change becomes incredibly tough to do.

Keep in thoughts, however, that via accepting your proper self and your cutting-edge situation, you aren't condemning yourself to permanently live together along with your troubles. This is a very common worry and can clearly save you us from moving ahead with our existence for plenty weeks, months, or maybe years.

State frivolously to your self: "I am wherein I am and that's good enough." Then u.S. Of america, "I am in which I am and that's good enough... however it doesn't imply that I need to stay proper here." Did you be aware the vibrational difference amongst the ones statements? Just the slightest, smallest shift to your notion can start to get the strength shifting that can assist propel us earlier. The EFT setup assertion is used solely to address psychological reversal.

Understand that self-popularity EFT affirmations will definitely can help you renowned and take transport of your self. These affirmations must be stated at the equal time as you are tapping as they artwork alongside every other. The first step toward self-elegance is changing the way you accept as true with you studied and address yourself, and it starts offevolved offevolved with the aid of way of first viewing your lifestyles in a one-of-a-type attitude. The subsequent step might be to make adjustments in your each day lifestyles - which you may do effects via figuring out the activities that you are feeling you maximum experience doing or ones which is probably most exceptional to cope with. Once you have got got were given a experience of the matters which you need to alternate you could begin thru imposing them for your each day hobby time table.

The special advantage of the use of a self-reputation EFT confirmation is that it'll will let you renowned and take transport of all of your emotions. This is an obvious step inside the recovery method and it's miles paramount to each state of affairs.

As all and sundry understand, maximum human beings hold onto awful feelings of their frame. These awful emotions ultimately start to have an impact on our ordinary fitness and health, inflicting us to emerge as sick or emotionally unbalanced. Usually, many human beings will at the least have a clue of what introduced approximately their infection, but maximum will no longer understand the fundamental purpose in their troubles. This can then bring about excessive results that can motive every physical and emotional ache. Sadly, maximum human beings definitely deny this is taking place to them with a view to maintain with their ordinary lives. However, what they fail to recognize is that, despite the fact that they have got managed to cover the ache, there still exists an energetic imbalance internal them. Unwittingly, they then create greater imbalances within them so as for his or her body to reap equilibrium. This maintains in a vicious cycle. In order to heal emotional ache, someone is needed to virtually accept him or herself with the useful resource of the use of searching after themselves and with the beneficial resource of being real to themselves. This can be finished with the aid of the use of in truth inviting to your conscious attention. Therefore, to heal emotional pain we need to first famend it.

Moreover, a self-recognition EFT confirmation requires that to be able to heal emotional pain you have to obtain your self for the worrying conditions which you have already endured. This approach that you need to no longer punish your self for the beyond, but as an alternative, examine the beyond as a gaining knowledge of revel in. Then forgive your self through way of letting move of those past studies. Since you deserve a glowing starting, it's miles important to widely recognized your feelings, so positioned them in the back of you, and then cherish what you have had been given placed from the ones challenges and respect the manner you controlled to conquer them.

An possibility thing to recollect whilst using EFT affirmations for self-beauty is which you have to honor what you are doing and take shipping of which you are doing the exceptional that you could with what you have got proper now. This manner that you want to renowned the achievements which you have had, however additionally to permit bypass the topics that you in no way did. Just endure in thoughts that achievement requires that you make development, so that you will although need to strive for added to come lower back.

Another self-popularity EFT affirmation calls for that one ought to discover ways to love, take transport of, and admire all components of him or herself. This way a person is precise in his or her very private manner and consequently one ought no longer to look at himself or herself to different human beings, as this may generate a lousy have an impact on about one's very own self. Consequently if we had been to faucet "I am gaining knowledge of to love, take transport of and appreciate all components of me" - the frame is privy to that this is actual because it's miles primarily based totally mostly on a notion and it fits the present day perception. This method that at the same time as tapping, one must constantly use high-quality phrases in the tapping affirmations.

However, in a few instances, this middle setup declaration might not artwork or the shift is virtually brief and the trouble continues on returning. In this form of state of affairs, setup statements which have been changed or extra extremely good will normally help in enhancing the tapping consequences. A few examples of advanced setup statements to address self-popularity encompass:

• I actually have the belief of accepting myself in line with my modern-day situation

• I additionally respect the feelings that I actually have currently

• I get hold of who I am and the way I experience

• I honor myself for a way difficult this is (has been)

• I deeply and simply be for the reason that I am doing the exquisite that I can

• I am reading to be ok with myself... truely as I am

• I honor and recognize myself for a way difficult this has been

• I am inclined to love and take delivery of myself anyway

• I thank, love and apprehend myself

• I am open to the concept of accepting myself simply the manner I am

• I take transport of all of me now, along with the emotions I actually have

Self-Actualization

This is some different gain of tapping in that it permits us to reveal our thoughts and feeling spherical and definitely open up. When our emotions and energy start to shift, and we are feeling more accepting of ourselves and the situation that we currently discover ourselves in, we are able to begin to upload in particular affirmations which is probably referred to as 'Turn Around' and 'Allowing' affirmations. These phrases are perfect to apply during the early ranges of tapping and you do now not sense comfortable however in the utilization of more potent or extra powerful affirmations.

Do be aware that in case you do come on too strong or try to flow into too speedy, your unconscious mind need to probable lock-up. This can be prevented by means of the use of the usage of actually asking questions and making opportunity statements with the intention to help rework the horrible power.

Whenever a Turn Around or Allowing declaration is established by the usage of our subconscious mind, we right now start to feel more snug and inclined to just go along with the drift of existence. As stated previously, each time we're in a resisting mind-set trade will now not be viable.

When your emotions are shifting and you are experiencing elegance of yourself and your modern-day-day scenario, this must seem quite with out issues and quick. It is critical to encompass Turn Around statements within the course of tapping on the way to let you do just that. These are very crucial statements to embody, specially during the early tapping manner with the intention to accept more affirmations which may be best.

However, it need to be stated that the ones must now not be performed too fast as it'd bring about the unconscious part of the mind locking up. Therefore, questions need to be finished so that you can permit a smooth transformation, and to prevent the method from being hindered in any way. If the ones remarkable and allowing statements are ordinary through the unconscious a part of the thoughts, you have to begin to enjoy more calm and cushty and therefore no resistance to exchange takes place. It is advocate that for tremendous consequences the wrist is tapped while saying the modern-day issue being skilled. Below are a few examples that you can use. As you take a look at thru them, be aware of how your body reacts to each of the statements. Practice some of them now through tapping your karate chop element and pronouncing the statements alongside side the modern hassle that you are managing right now.

• I will find out a way through this by means of some means

• I am open to locating a one in all a kind way to check this

• I permit my thoughts and frame to assist me remedy this

• I permit myself to move through this at the high-quality pace for me

• I am starting to sense that I can permit this skip

If any of these statements are stated whilst tapping, the unconscious a part of the mind knows that it is proper; but horrible statements ought to in no manner be covered on the equal time as tapping due to the fact the subconscious can't differentiate between high great and lousy statements.

Making a Decision and Taking the First Step

Dr. Pat Carrington is an EFT professional that created a totally effective EFT technique called the EFT Choices Method. Adding choice, or choice statements, into the tapping affirmations can absolutely useful useful resource us in focusing better on our intentions and dreams, even as simultaneously enhancing our regular tapping consequences.

In order to make those kinds of terms as effective as possible, it's miles vital to select a word that reasons the unconscious thoughts to at once suppose which you are moving too rapid, or that you couldn't however be organized to cope with this word or scenario.

That being stated, however, if we experience a "Yeah, however..." or a tail-ender unexpectedly nipping in the lower back of our minds at the same time as tapping on a selected choices phrase, that is a tremendous indicator that you could in all likelihood need to step decrease returned and try to deal with this hassle from a one-of-a-type thoughts-set.

On the alternative hand, tail-enders can be quite valuable. In maximum times, those tail-enders in reality show clues to us about why we are feeling caught and now not able to obtain our desires and intentions. As rapid as this records emerges, along with unprocessed emotions or newly placed beliefs, you want to start to tap on it.

If it is not your motive proper now to discover any tail-enders, then previous to tapping with a robust effective EFT confirmation, it is vital to apprehend whether or no longer you have got shifted the terrible energies effectively. If, as an opportunity, you've got were given have been given been truely · making assumptions and function failed to test your EFT artwork, then there may be a outstanding threat that you could wind up losing every your treasured time and your try.

The EFT Temporal Tap is one such technique that falls into the magnificence of 'it's higher to realize first'. You definitely do now not want to turn out to be with painful temples and no treatment or excessive quality exchange in sight.

Do be conscious that in case you experience any resistance even as you're tapping with strong high pleasant statements that it's miles pleasant to change up the terms a bit. For example, the phrase "I've determined to..." may be changed to kingdom "I am open to the possibility of..."

Some of the EFT Choices tapping affirmations embody:

• I really have determined to start to allow this hassle pass

- I honestly have determined to take it absolutely in the future at a time

- I pick out out to feel comfortable and non violent

- I pick out out to be at peace with this in a manner that works splendid for me

- I pick out to permit myself to heal in a manner that works fine for me

- I actually have decided to reclaim my non-public strength

- I without a doubt have decided to loosen up and revel in at peace, proper here, right now

- I truly have decided to be greater open and accepting regarding this hassle

- I select to be okay with this, in a way that works top notch for me

- I reclaim my revel in of personal protection proper right here, proper now

- I pick to discover new methods to artwork this hassle out

Just like any other techniques of confirmation, the tapping method is going hand in hand with pronouncing any of those terms.

Many humans in recent times are better at wondering and running subjects out in their heads than they're in figuring out their emotions and the sensations they may be experiencing inner their our bodies.

If you find out that you are this type of humans and are having a hard time getting into touch collectively with your frame eventually of EFT, the very quality element to do is try to loosen up and actually go along with the tapping technique. Fake it 'til you're making it! After a while, the link amongst your mind and your body will reactivate.

Some EFT practitioners suggest doing one or rounds of EFT, repeating every set up phrase three times consistent with meridian issue in step with round.

Next, you can do some greater rounds the usage of a reminder assertion. These rounds typically occur even as the number one round or of following the tapping series and citing the affirmations has not cleared up the issue to hand. A reminder announcement is best a quick word or a word that first-class explains the hassle and that you state aloud each time you faucet one of the meridian elements in the EFT tapping series. By doing so, you're continually 'reminding' your thoughts and frame about the trouble you're presently taking walks on, or walking through because the case may be.

One of the exquisite varieties of reminder statements to lease is individuals who resemble the statement you selected for your preliminary confirmation. However, you could boost up this method even extra with the resource of honestly substituting a word or brief phrase in desire to a whole declaration sentence.

For instance, if you have been trying to conquer your addiction to meals, your set up assertion could likely study:

"Even despite the fact that I am hooked on food, I deeply and genuinely receive myself."

With this affirmation the reminder phase could encompass the phrases 'hooked on food'. Simply reciting this reminder word, alongside aspect the immoderate superb confirmation, can help you to better address your hassle.

Chapter 10: Eft Tapping For Weight Loss And Inner Peace

Tapping for weight reduction is based totally mostly on the precept that weight benefit and overeating, collectively with the cravings we get for food, is rooted in tension. Through its use to alleviate tension and stress, tapping lets in address this problem, and here is why.

Our emotional united states of america has a tremendous impact on our urge for food, our digestive device, and the manner we keep the strength that comes from our meals. Stress remedy is essential for staying healthier and higher in form as well, for accelerated pressure tiers trigger the release of the hormone cortisol in higher tiers. What does cortisol do in terms of weight benefit? It collects fats in the course of the midriff, which poses a big scientific threat for the development of weight problems and diabetes.

That being stated, how can we reign in our feelings, lower cravings, and analyze no longer to get so labored up about starvation or fullness via tapping? This exercise will help you determine via weight reduction issues and acquire inner peace.

EFT Working Towards Overcoming Bad Eating Habits

Let's face it, occasionally you notice a food which you understand to be scrumptious, and also you truly want it for the flavor! Many instances, you can fight this feel, but have you ever ever begun to increase an actual hunger to your belly on the equal time as seeing part of meals that tastes proper?

The identical technological facts takes vicinity close to substance abuse. What's taking region right right here is that there can be a highbrow and emotional reaction to seeing food or your selected drink this is tricking you into believing you are hungry or thirsty. Are you hungry? Are you thirsty? Maybe, but probable no longer. Something inside you is telling you which you need that slice of pizza and you want to scrub it down with a bottle of your selected beer. You do not, so what is going on?

Sometimes it's far an trouble of fulfilment, a yearning for something that is being projected onto the food, or a need for comfort and in our case, it is the divorce that brings your longing out.

The trick is to be aware, and in being conscious, you could discover extra powerful terms to use at some stage in your tapping carrying sports activities. Tune into the manner you sense if you have a yearning or discover your frame is telling you it's far hungry or thirsty despite the fact that you in reality ate or had a bottle or of beer.

Are you feeling like if you do now not consume that particular slice of pizza, you will omit out on the particular taste of that pizza? Do you worry you may be thinking about it all day in case you do not consume it? How about this – are you in a 2nd of strain, seeking out a distraction, and experience that having a few aspect to devour or drink in significant may also make you revel in higher?

A word like this could tackle an problem of comfort: "Even even though I really need that slice of pizza, I recognize I just need comfort at the same time as you bear in mind that I even have no longer visible my buddies in a while or I do now not have a person to love me anymore." Or, for tension or misery, you can use "I realise I really want to shop for the vodka they are promoting over there, but I recognize I'm virtually feeling impulsive thinking about I've already spent a lot time on my own nowadays." Try to bear in mind what's taking vicinity in tandem at the side of your hunger – temper stresses, feeling crushed, trying to flavor some aspect familiar, or feeling lonely.

The element is that this: almost about weight reduction, don't forget the way you feel to redirect your electricity. You can stay with phrases like "Even even though I'm feeling worn-out, I may be satisfied I went to the fitness center and labored out tough," it is simply as useful to start on the supply of the problem.

Be Aware of Hunger and Fullness

This is vital, because it will impact even as you begin tapping. It's always a excellent concept to price the depth of your hunger in advance than you even start the workout, so you understand at the equal time as it's miles vital to do something high quality approximately it.

Also, to supplement your tapping, it's an notable concept to stick to a habitual approximately while you consume, how a whole lot water you may drink, and what styles of food you may paintings to hold out of the residence to keep you at the right music. Will you eat 3 huge meals a day without snacking, or will you unfold out your food consumption into six small food an afternoon? A accurate manner to parent out an powerful plan is to reveal how regularly you legitimately feel hungry, and to test out for substances you typically generally tend to eat the most customarily.

Once you have received a few perception into your skip-to materials and the frequency of cravings, paintings around it! Always go through in mind to be prlvy to how you experience when you have a craving, and widely known if you have some problem looming over you that is developing cravings or whether or not a few component critical simply occurred this is inflicting an increase on your appetite.

Follow Through with The Intensity Scale

Keep a sharp eye on how intense your hunger is. What you may think is a 6 or 7 on the size of depth for the manner you're feeling, may probable best be a 2 or a three even as positioned into mindset, counting on how severe you allow your hunger get.

It's normally an incredible rule of thumb to consume on the same time as you're hungry, however in case you find out yourself continuously craving for food when you need to now not be, it is time to start searching on the symptoms to your life.

Are you eating properly? Do you consume meals which may be addicting, or which might be so excessive in taste that they may be tough to place away? Can you wait 5 mins to devour? Could you push it to 15 minutes? How loads longer should you go with out food with out feeling pain? Don't push your self into distress, however those are questions you have to ask yourself to determine whether you are hungry, having a craving, or avoiding an underlying problem of tension or pressure that might be a higher consciousness of your tapping.

Tapping Sequence and Statements for Energy

Step One: Find Your Unconscious Blocks

Begin through absolutely writing out your precise weight loss cause. This might also need to suggest which you write what number of kilos you want to lose, the manner you would really like to experience, and the way your life goes to appearance while you gain that goal. This is what your aware purpose is.

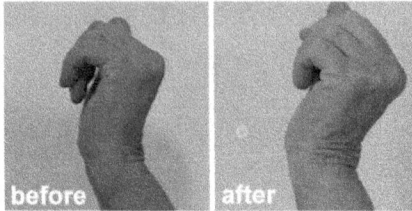

'Any sufficiently advanced technology is indistinguishable from magic.'
Arthur C. Clarke

Lack of mobility from **arthritis** before .. and after one minute

As you write down your intention, you may enjoy terrible feelings and thoughts. These regularly get up as "yeah, but..." and may be a tremendous impediment or block earlier than you acquire your purpose. Common issues near weight reduction are, "Yeah, but there may be no manner I might be capable of preserve my reason weight", "I'm already too worn-out, and this may take too much artwork", "I've by no means been able to shed pounds in advance than, why will this be any special?" and so on.

Write the ones horrific ideals down and rate them on a scale of 0 to ten. A 10 would probable mean it's miles the maximum intense or real for you at that modern-day-day second. You are going to be re-rating these items after some tapping rounds. The intention is to get those numbers to lower, and you faucet until it does.

Step Two: Get Rid of Your Blocks

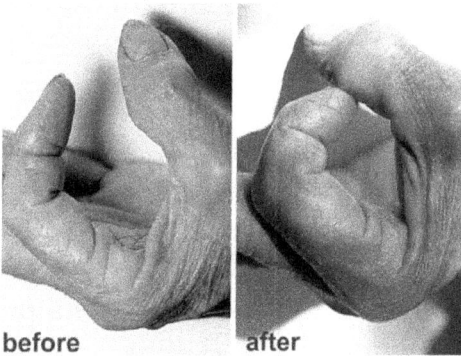

before   after

This is at the same time as you start your tapping. This is a pattern script that you could use, enjoy free to alternate it to suit your problems, and if, at the equal time as you're tapping, you revel in such as you want to say some thing other than what you had deliberate, allow it take place. If a phrase comes up that you did now not count on, or have planned, say it due to the fact you possibly need to address that hassle. Let this broaden organically.

Begin through way of tapping the karate chop element and say, "despite the fact that I even have loads to do, I'm worn-out and overwhelmed... I cannot upload a few thing else to my time desk, and it is probably too much... I nonetheless take shipping of and love myself." Do this three times.

Begin tapping thru the alternative factors, beginning with the internal eye to the top of the pinnacle. Here are a few matters you may say.

? Inner eye: I already do an excessive amount of.

? Outer eye: I'm not able to do the whole lot.

? Under eye: It's going to be an excessive amount of artwork and too hard.

? Chin: I already enjoy overwhelmed, and I am not capable of function some thing else to my time desk.

? Collarbone: I do no longer need to do some thing else.

? Underarm: I sense in reality crushed.

? Top of head: This is going to be too tough, and I won't be able to do it.

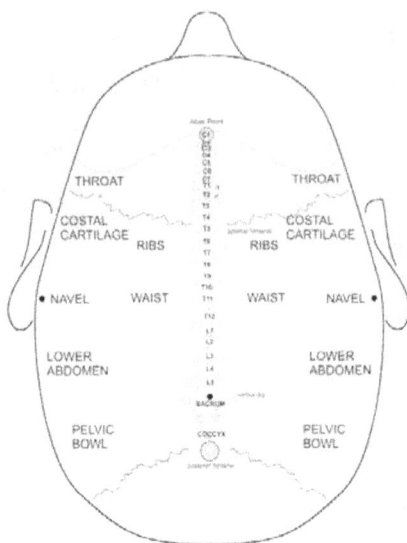

Continue to try this until your feelings begin to shift, or you may examine the shift and keep to faucet. You will turn out to be tapping via the ones elements severa instances, and you will in all likelihood change what you assert at every factor severa instances to cope with your shifting viewpoints. You also can use awesome possibilities such because it's not every other weight loss plan that restricts, forces, gets rid of favored meals, or counting electricity. Neither is it an workout plan, but rather, it is a letting technique and accepting and loving yourself tool as nicely.

After more than one tapping rounds, you should forestall and fee the doubts you had written down in advance. Once your rankings have reduced significantly, otherwise you enjoy like you have got blanketed as loads as you may on your first consultation, then you can prevent. In one week come once more and examine over the ones doubts and your weight loss plans. See what feelings rise up, and price the doubts. Do extra tapping in case you experience you need to, which you need to in case you price anything about a 3.

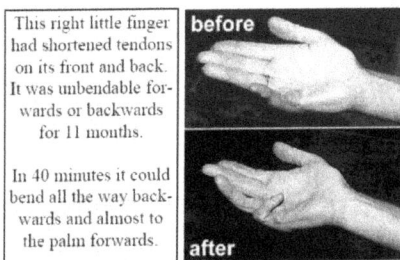

| This right little finger had shortened tendons on its front and back. It was unbendable for-wards or backwards for 11 months. | before |
| In 40 minutes it could bend all the way back-wards and almost to the palm forwards. | after |

EFT Tapping for Our Emotions

EFT is a powerful tool that assist you to recognize more about your self, your strengths and your weaknesses. It permit you to overcome emotional problems and beautify relationships.

Before we get began, permit me remind you that this e-book is not supposed as an alternative for the scientific advice of certified physicians.

Relationship Issues

One of the critical wishes of all of us is to be loved. When a person feels that he or she is not noted and feels unloved, it in reality creates dating problems, depression and low conceitedness.

We have a herbal tendency to be attracted to others who've similar persona tendencies.

For example, if you fee honesty, you are much more likely to draw and be interested by an honest man or woman. If you adore your self, you will then be much more likely to satisfy and appeal to others closer to you which might be at the identical vibration or frequency.

However, in case you hate your self, then you actually are growing obstacles that save you others from getting close to you and getting into your lifestyles. Negative emotions, which encompass jealousy, can severely damage private relationships and wishes to be addressed.

If you revel in that you are jealous or harbor any horrible mind both toward yourself or your accomplice, then it is most probable that the ones thoughts or emotions also are hurting your relationship. The first step to addressing the ones problems is to take ownership of them.

Whether you've got troubles getting close to someone, want to move away a dating, address jealousy, anger or some other negative emotion, then you may comply with the steps under.

Tapping Script for Relationship Issues

Below are examples of setup scripts you may use for the tapping manner. Feel loose to adjust them, in reality in order that they in shape and reflect your personal desires.

Even despite the fact that I am afraid of getting near, I take delivery of my flaws and myself and could have the capacity to conquer the ones problems.

Even despite the fact that I had abusive relationships within the beyond, I acquire that I can be a better partner and will grasp braveness.

Even although I get jealous, I love and take shipping of myself completely.

Next, faucet for your energy meridian factors, beginning with the karate chop component (it's the element of your hand) after which transferring down from the top, whilst reciting your phrase.

Repeat the method and check the way you feel. Do you experience less jealous? Are you greater snug in the relationship? If you want to, you may repeat the manner.

Dealing with Personal Differences In A Relationship

When you're in a relationship, there are often pretty some non-public problems that arise that you'll want to take care of, for each you and your companion.

Spending brilliant time together and talking openly approximately non-public variations permit you to triumph over notable obstacles within the dating.

Tapping Procedure to Deal with Personal Differences

? Both of you need to sit down down together and list down the coolest capabilities you want to your associate.

? Next, write down the tendencies you do now not like on your companion. I'm conscious that this can be tough, but it's far remarkable, to be honest.

? Then, write down what opinions for your dating made you sense the happiest (as an instance, surprise items).

? Now, you need to speak along with your associate approximately what you wrote down, emphasizing the coolest traits and being sincere about the terrible.

? Formulate setup phrases like "Even even though I revel in lonely even as he is at artwork, I apprehend that he loves me" or "Even despite the fact that we argue, I recognize that she loves me." It is an notable exercise to start with a minor trouble.

? You may also moreover save you the machine thru tapping collectively. You can also use tapping scripts like "We love each particular, and we are able to artwork collectively on our flaws."

Chapter 11: Tug Testing™ For

Your Water Level

As you may be conscious, the water degree for your frame rises while the moon gets entire, and drops in a moonless sky. No moon, some moon, complete moon. Relaxed, energetic, balanced. Alternatively, sluggish, hyperactive, spun out. This depends on how loads water you have got got in addition to how properly you direct the restrained water you have got on your frame.

It's broadly recognized that the quantity of water on your frame is a first-rate determinant of your fitness. You are nicely while the water to your nicely is entire and no longer sloshing spherical an excessive amount of—without a doubt flowing nicely.

Naturally, you also are probably to stay longer. Did you recognize that a infant's body is 90% water? An man or woman's frame is 70% water. You may be horrified to realise that an vintage person's body is typically simplest 60% water. Now, irrespective of your age, you can boom the water ranges for your body yet again, and distribute them evenly. It enables to regenerate your cells so that you stay a longer, greater healthy lifestyles with lots much less pain.

You'll find out that if a slight tug of your hair or pores and skin strengthens your breath-ing it indicates which you need greater water. So tug your hair gently at the yet again of your head and test your respiratory. If your in breath and out breath begin to your tummy it famous that 'Yes, that a part of my face wishes more natural water'.

In factor of reality, the again of your scalp relates to your face's want for water. The left issue of your scalp pertains to the left component of your body. And the proper element of your scalp relates to the right facet of your frame's need for water. Only whilst all 3 places make you begin your inside and out breath for your chest—that is, while Tummy Testing™ says 'No extra, thanks' - is your frame complete of water. This wondrous tool for self trying out is referred to as Tug Testing™.

Watch it carefully. Do you understand that you can placed the water into your frame and permit it out yet again with out using all of it, leaving a few cells dry and beneath functioning?

Or you can ensure that every one components of your frame have ok hydration thru Tug Testing™, step by step, at some point of your scalp. And you can stability the water stages to your body by using way of setting the BLUE (-) face of your D Everlasting Décolletage Smoother™ in your navel to preserve the Everlasting Cream 'Water ranges balance now'. Please look at the Scalp Reflexology™ chart, confirmed on the following web web page, for extra one-of-a-kind element.

Additionally, you could additionally Tug Test™ for meals, sleep, deep rest and lots of unique vital elements of your herbal manner of existence. Look up your Scalp Reflexology™ chart, find out what you want and do it!

Arthritis with loss of hand closure in advance than … and with closure after

The Tug Test™

Test the water diploma in every a part of your body. Tug your hair gently. If Tummy Testing™ says 'Yes' you want greater water within the related a part of your body.

Prevention of Dehydration

You see, the not unusual person loses between and three litres of water an afternoon thru the breath, sweat, and urine. This number can speedy growth or lower based totally absolutely really on the types of physical or highbrow sports that someone en-gages in. Heavy exercising can cause a body to lose more than 2 litres an hour! To save you dehydration you without a doubt need to pinnacle off the liquids which is probably misplaced during the day. Many assets and internet web sites will inform you to drink eight glasses of water an afternoon, or come up with a set amount of litres to drink however the sincere fact is that each BODY is great and best you will recognise how masses your BODY dreams.

Naturally, nice YOU can comprehend how lots water YOU want to be at your top notch. That's right, herbal WATER. Not soda, not juice, now not sugar-drinks. Pay interest in your fluid loss and purpose to pinnacle off it as it's far being misplaced. By the time you sense simply thirsty you're already stricken by dehydration - you in truth want to keep away from turning into thirsty inside the first vicinity. Pay interest to the coloration of your urine as darkish urine is mostly a traditional indicator that you are dehydrated.

The Causes of Dehydration

It actually so happens that there are various matters that might cause dehydration, the maximum commonplace are vomiting, diarrhea, blood loss, malnutrition, and undeniable antique failure to top off essential liquids out of place from sweating and urination (now not consuming enough water). Many commonplace ailments and illnesses can cause acute dehydration due to the prolonged frame temperature and sweating that commonly get up. This is why you want to drink plenty of fluids at the equal time as you are ill. Your body makes use of fluids to expel pollutants similarly to to maintain your device flexible, lubricated and on foot without difficulty.

The Signs and Symptoms of Dehydration

I want to tell you that signs of dehydration usually begin with thirst and development to extra alarming manifestations due to the truth the want for water will become extra dire. The preliminary telltale signs and symptoms and symptoms and symptoms and signs and symptoms of slight dehydration in adults seem while the frame has misplaced approximately 2% of it's far favored fluid. These slight dehydration signs and symptoms and signs and symptoms are regularly (but no longer restricted to) thirst, dry pores and skin, loss of urge for meals, dry mouth, pores and pores and skin flushing, darkish colored urine, fatigue or weak point, chills, and head rushes.

If the dehydration is authorized to maintain unabated, while the entire fluid loss reaches five% the subsequent effects of dehydration are normally skilled:

• Increased coronary heart price

• Increased respiration

- Decreased sweating

- Decreased urination

- Increased body temperature

- Extreme fatigue

- Muscle cramps

- Headaches

- Nausea

- Tingling of the limbs

Can you understand that once the body in the end reaches 10% fluid loss, emergency help is favored IMMEDIATELY! 10% fluid loss and above is regularly lethal! Symptoms of extreme dehydration include:

- Muscle spasms

- Vomiting

- Racing pulse

- Shrivelled skin

- Dim imaginative and prescient

- Painful urination

- Confusion

- Difficulty respiratory

- Seizures

- Chest and Abdominal ache

- Unconsciousness

As I've referred to, signs of dehydration will variety from individual to person due to the truth the body is a complicated community of incorporated structures and all of us's frame is terrific. When those structures are disturbed because of lack of fluids there might be numerous not unusual symptoms and symptoms and symptoms shared with the aid of most our our bodies, however there can also be unusual or surprising responses. Signs of dehydration in a child will no longer be much like the ones professional through a youngster, adult or inside the aged. Ultimately, reliable dehydration prevention is the fantastic treatment for each age organization from 0 to a hundred and twenty and past.

Treatment for Dehydration

Of direction, while someone turns into dehydrated they have got furthermore lost electrolytes so it's miles very vital to fill up them along factor the natural water. The sort of essential electrolytes wanted for rehydration are sodium and potassium salts normally positioned in seaweed. Vital electrolytes are wanted for electro-chemical reactions inside healthy cells. A lack of electrolytes in the frame can interfere with the chemical reactions wanted for wholesome mobile operation and is referred to as water intoxication. This can grow to be a crucial scenario and has led to dying in immoderate times.

Straight up, if a person is showing minor signs and signs and signs and symptoms, deliver them hundreds of water and allow them to drink it very slowly, in small, clean sips. Electrolytes are also observed in salty substances but ingesting any meals at the same time as dehydrated will most effective dehydrate the frame extra for the reason that fluids are required for digestion. Slowly pinnacle off the body's beverages with water and study that up, after symptoms and signs and symptoms have subsided, with a small salty snack collectively with miso soup with seaweed or a very mild meal.

Watch it carefully due to the reality if someone is displaying some of the more immoderate signs and signs of dehydration, and past the factor in which ingestion of the right fluids will assist, it's best to get medical interest right now.

Treatment for Chronically Dry Skin

Did you ever recognize that your pores and pores and skin can even though be jarringly dry even while you drink a number of water because it is going to remarkable elements of your body? You need to open the capillary sphincters on your pores and skin to get the blood flowing into your ravenous pores and skin cells. If your pores and pores and pores and skin is dry, its due to the fact its cells are starved of hydration. The water isn't flowing thru on your cells.

What I'm saying is, offer your self the subsequent Everlasting Creams in a triple technique:

"Skin rejuvenates abruptly now"

"Skin moisturises now"

"Diaphragm relaxes abruptly now"

Significantly, this components assists the rehydration of your dermis - the top layer of your pores and skin. You examine extra approximately it and its excellent use at your Cleopatra Skin Face Lift Yoga seminar.

I'm afraid that ingesting caffeine dries out your skin due to the fact it's far a diuretic. This manner that the water in your cup of tea or coffee goes into your bloodstream then immediately from your kidneys in advance than it reaches your impoverished pores and pores and skin cells.

Come to reflect onconsideration on it, caffeine takes area in tea (which includes green tea), coffee, cocoa, cacao, chocolate, cola and guarana.

Diuretic and Non-Diuretic Herbs

Smoking reasons wrinkles and sag

You'll be amazed to comprehend why wrinkles shape. Read on.

Believe it or no longer enzymes known as matrix metallaproteinases (MMPs) break up the fibres that form collagen in your frame. It's the connective tissue that makes up round 50% of pores and pores and skin.

Smoking will boom MMP production so more of your collagen is damaged down. And it decreases the manufacturing of smooth collagen by means of using manner of 40%. A wrinkle is a depletion of tissue. So is osteoporosis ("pores or holes within the bones")

If you smoke, you'll have an lousy lot much less collagen, because of this that that greater wrinkle formation and extra sag. And brittle bones.

Fluoride reasons wrinkles and sag

You can gain extensively, proper now, from understanding what to drink.

It in order that takes region that 25% of number one tranquillisers are related with fluoride so eating natural, non-fluoridated water sharpens your mind.

Be very careful. Fluoridated populations are extra docile and obedient. This includes cattle. And fluoridated cities show no massive improvement in increase-ing dental decay.

What's more, fluoridation has been definitely rejected in Denmark. Sweden and most European nations banned it because of feasible renal and neuromuscular damage and shocking little one mortality.

Fluoridation may additionally purpose dental fluorosis - an unpleasant mottling of your enamel.

I've were given to tell you, but, that in New Zealand, statistics showed greater upgrades in dental health (a whole lot tons less dental decay) in non-fluoridated in preference to fluoridated areas. In Tucson, Arizona, studies confirmed that the more fluoride an harmless toddler drank, the more cavities appeared of their teeth. Other research showed multiplied prevalence of hip fractures and bone most cancers. Astounding!

Similarly, fluoride disrupts the synthesis of collagen and ends in its damage-down in bone, tendon, muscle, cartilage, lungs, kidneys, trachea and pores and skin. Your pores and skin is eighty% collagen, so fluoride reasons telltale wrinkles!!

As most humans recognize, processed food containing water (together with fruit juice or canned peas) furthermore consists of fluoride.

It is extensively recognized that boiling water does now not dispose of fluoride. It concentrates it thru putting off the water. It's splendid that distilled water is fluoride unfastened.

The reality of the trouble is that you want to train your self further so why no longer go to www.Healthful-communications.Com or are seeking the internet for brilliant interesting statistics about fluoride. Then you could determine for your self.

Chapter 12: The Basic Recipe For Weight Loss

The essential EFT "recipe" consists of the subsequent 4 steps, for you to be mentioned in detail inside the subsequent chapters:

Step 0 - Drink water

Step 1 - Tune in and charge

Close your eyes. Take a deep breath as you've got a study your whole body for any tightness or bodily pain. On a scale of zero to 10 (zero being "no pain" and ten being "worst ache"), how will I price my emotional ache?

The technique to this question can be the rating that you can use as a baseline. Keep in mind that the greater element you have about your pain, the higher your probabilities of making EFT give you the consequences you need.

Step 2 – Clearing of intellectual reversal

Psychologically reversed is a situation wherein the active problem that surrounds the precise vicinity wherein the hassle takes place is reversed.

To perform mental reversal for weight loss troubles, tap the area with red dots inside the picture beneath ("karate factor"). You may additionally choose the hand, which feels more cushty for you. Use the four palms of your dominant hand to tap on the dotted area of the opportunity hand. Tap approximately 7 seconds for every assertion. Continue tapping until you have were given completed pronouncing all the following statements:

• In spite of being overweight, I attain myself sincerely, I though love and certainly take transport of myself.

• In spite of being overweight, I forgive myself for a few element I in reality have completed to contribute to the ache.

• In spite of being obese, I forgive the alternative people who've introduced to my pain

• In spite of being overweight, I will all the time love and truely take transport of myself.

REPEAT PSYCHOLOGICAL REVERSAL THREE TIMES. Make tremendous which you say the statements aloud and energetically, as even though what the statements imply are in reality real irrespective of the truth which you do now not really consider them. I realise it can every so often be hard to mention some aspect that you do no longer actually accept as true with in. However, without a doubt

take delivery of as genuine with inside the method and you can in the end sense for your coronary coronary heart which you are starting to just accept as actual with the ones statements. However, you may say the statements silently or thru manner of heart as you breathe.

Step three – Tap

Here are the stairs in tapping. Tap approximately 7 seconds on each of the factors.

1. Tap on the number one aspect at the same time as announcing the four statements. Continue tapping till you've got got said all statements.

2. Go to and faucet the second component even as announcing the 4 statements.

three. Repeat the tapping and the statements till you have got completed all eight elements.

4. After you've got finished, inhale and exhale deeply.

5. Drink simply sufficient water.

Start tapping your index and center palms at the tapping elements of your body:

1. Eyebrow point, that is placed closest to the inner stop of your left eyebrow. Do ensure despite the fact that, that you do

no longer pass all of the manner right down to your nostril's bridge.

• In spite of being overweight, I however love and virtually take shipping of myself.

• In spite of being overweight, I forgive myself for whatever I definitely have carried out to make contributions to the pain.

• In spite of being overweight, I forgive the opposite humans who have introduced to my ache

• In spite of being obese, I will for all time love and completely take delivery of myself.

2. Side-of-the-eye factor, that is placed closest to the outside end of your right eye. Make remarkable that you do not poke your eyeball. If you abruptly be aware that your imaginative and prescient started out to grow to be blurred otherwise you spot a flash of moderate or

darkness, it way that the wrong spot is being tapped.

• In spite of being obese, I however love and in fact take delivery of myself.

• In spite of being obese, I forgive myself for some thing I surely have performed to make contributions to the pain.

• In spite of being overweight, I forgive the alternative humans who have added to my pain

• In spite of being obese, I will for all time love and surely get hold of myself.

3. Under-the-eye element, it's miles located for your left cheekbone sincerely below your student. If you have got sinusitis, you can select to tap very lightly.

• In spite of being obese, I despite the truth that love and completely take shipping of myself.

• In spite of being obese, I forgive myself for some thing I genuinely have accomplished to contribute to the ache.

• In spite of being obese, I forgive the opposite people who have brought to my ache

• In spite of being overweight, I will all the time love and certainly take shipping of myself.

4. Under-the-nose issue, this is located precisely among your nose and your pinnacle lip.

• In spite of being overweight, I nevertheless love and simply take delivery of myself.

• In spite of being obese, I forgive myself for a few thing I even have finished to make a contribution to the pain.

• In spite of being obese, I forgive the possibility human beings who've delivered to my ache

• In spite of being obese, I will all of the time love and surely acquire myself.

five. Under-the-mouth issue, that is placed at the dip that connects your chin and reduce lip.

• In spite of being obese, I although love and genuinely take shipping of myself.

• In spite of being overweight, I forgive myself for some difficulty I even have done to make a contribution to the ache.

• In spite of being overweight, I forgive the possibility people who've delivered to my pain

• In spite of being obese, I will all the time love and in reality receive myself.

6. Collarbone issue, that is positioned exactly wherein your collarbone and your sternum meet.

• In spite of being overweight, I though love and definitely accumulate myself.

• In spite of being overweight, I forgive myself for a few thing I actually have finished to make contributions to the pain.

• In spite of being obese, I forgive the possibility people who have introduced to my ache

• In spite of being obese, I will forever love and in reality take shipping of myself.

7. Under-the-arm element, this is positioned on the difficulty of your body that is closer the lower again thing than the the front – round four inches down your armpit. If you poke your arms within the vicinity, you may locate it due to the fact the most clean element. To be which you are tapping on the right spot, use all your 4 fingers even as you faucet at the underneath-the-arm element.

• In spite of being obese, I but love and surely take transport of myself.

- In spite of being overweight, I forgive myself for something I truly have accomplished to contribute to the ache.

- In spite of being overweight, I forgive the alternative people who've brought to my ache

- In spite of being obese, I will all the time love and absolutely obtain myself.

eight. Top-of-the-head factor, it's far the peak or most factor on the pinnacle of your head.

- In spite of being obese, I nevertheless love and sincerely take shipping of myself.

- In spite of being obese, I forgive myself for a few element I virtually have done to make contributions to the pain.

- In spite of being overweight, I forgive the opportunity humans who have added to my pain

• In spite of being obese, I will all of the time love and truly take shipping of myself.

Step four – Tune in and re-rate

Inhale and exhale deeply. Also, take some other sip of water. When you are prepared, song in to the thing of emotional ache over again and ask the following questions:

• Did the intensity of the pain decrease, increase, or live the identical?

• Did any photo, imaginative and prescient, or idea entered your thoughts on the equal time as you have been tapping the outstanding frame elements? Were there any memory or character you remembered? If you replied "certain" to any of these questions, a few thing entered your mind is probably related to the pain which you are currently walking on.

• Rate the manner you enjoy now the use of the same scale of 0 to ten.

Chapter 13: Tips For Emotional Freedom Tapping

• While it's now not continually required to be simply particular along side your tapping, you need to virtually awareness at the language. Be specific and avoid broadstrokes whilst you're looking to address your issues.

• Try to pinpoint specific activities in which you advanced the conduct you want to address. If you have got have been given a fear of the dark, what started out out it? If you are terrified of snakes, grow to be there a selected occasion in your teenagers that introduced about your worry? Once you manage to outline it, try to take a look at your feelings spherical that occasion and smooth your emotions spherical it.

• Focus on the muse of your hassle. If you have got a fear of flying, is the worry coming from no longer being on pinnacle of things? Of being inside the middle of crowds? Again, it all boils right right down to the specifics of the trouble.

• Once you have got got your particular problems recognized, artwork on them one after the other. Measure their gravity and intensity to decide the collection of the manner you can deal with every one. Single out extra extreme problems and rank them consequently. What you need to do is maintain track of your development and keep score as you address the problem.

• Focus at the terrible. Remember that the cause is to recognize and well known the awful components so you can well pick out them and do something first rate about it. Emotional freedom approach works thru manner of clearing out the horrific emotions inherent to your emotional properly-being. Once you have got got mastered the emotions surrounding those, you could interest on doing some element to update the absence of negativity in your existence, this is wherein a bolstered assertion of positivity is to be had in.

• Write down a listing of your personal terrible activities that can have impacted your lifestyles in this form of way that it has skewed your perception and inherent herbal tendencies. Some examples encompass phobias, fears, judgments— the ones are all of the basis of lengthy-fame reactions that we've got as an individual. Write it all down on a listing— it's regular to have almost a list of 100.

• Don't surrender with out troubles. It took time to construct all the ones terrible feelings, in order that they received't continually be addressed in a single quick emotional freedom method tapping consultation. Do this constantly, frequently and with a clear and high-quality outlook. Give your self time to work in your issues and troubles. Be constant and preserve tapping. Changes can be subtle as a superb deal as they will be drastic and lifestyles-changing.

• While it's far possible to behavior a tapping consultation in public, it's far quality to gain this in personal. Find a cushty region wherein you could sit down down and be quiet collectively with your thoughts, wherein you can be your self and wherein you obtained't be involved with external elements. This can be your personal room or inside the privateness of your private rest room.

• Cut your self off. Not actually honestly through maintaining your self locked away for your personal non-public place however additionally through the use of using turning off your computer, your mobile devices or something else that could distract you from the hobby. Remember that all it takes is a couple of minutes from your day.

• Keep yourself hydrated. The complete thing of the exercise is to help you smooth out your terrible emotions,which can be finished extra correctly with water. Not to say that it takes a toll on you physical and anecdotal evidence notes how most folks that behavior tapping commonly generally tend to experience very thirsty after.

• Time yourself—set an alarm for 20 mins to half of an hour. You can in reality do this longer than 30 minutes if you may, however the proper might be around 20 to half-hour. Less than the allotted time technique you can now not enjoy the highbrow outcomes that you are focused on; greater than that and following the advocated time, you can now take pleasure on this experience of getting been able to cope with a protracted-fame emotional trouble.

www.ingramcontent.com/pod-product-compliance
Lightning Source LLC
Chambersburg PA
CBHW060233030426
42335CB00014B/1428